Table of Contents

Order this book from :

PRITCHETT & HULL ASSOCIATES, INC.
3440 OAKCLIFF RD NE STE 110
ATLANTA GA 30340-3006

or call toll free: 800-241-4925

2016 edition
Copyright© 1991, 1993, 1998,
2005, 2012, 2013, 2015
by Pritchett & Hull Associates, Inc.
All rights reserved. No part of this book
may be photocopied, reprinted or otherwise
reproduced without written permission from
Pritchett & Hull Associates, Inc.

Published and distributed by:
Pritchett & Hull Associates, Inc.

Printed in the U.S.A.

This book is only to help you learn,
and should not be used to replace any
advice or treatment from your health
care team.

To keep the text simple we often refer
to your child as "he/him."

Help your child help himself

Your child is one of many children who have asthma. Someday, he'll be able to manage his asthma without your help. But for now, it's up to you to take charge of his treatment and help him learn how to manage his asthma.

The best way to do this is with a treatment plan made just for him. This book will help you, your child and his doctor:

- **know what triggers** (causes) your child's asthma **flare-ups**

- **learn how to prevent and treat** his **flare-ups**

- **set up an asthma action plan** just for him

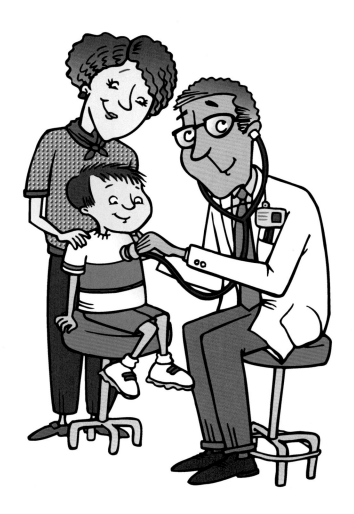

Asking for help

When you are not with your child, he may be shy about asking for help. Teach him that it's OK to tell other adults about triggers he needs to avoid or when he's having a flare-up.

What is asthma?

Asthma is a chronic (long-term) disease of the airways in the lungs. It's not catching, but it tends to run in families (inherited).

Your child may go for several weeks, months or even years with no symptoms or signs of asthma and then have a flare-up of coughing, wheezing, shortness of breath. **Even when he's not having symptoms, he is not cured.** He still has asthma. So continue to follow his treatment plan.

Normal breathing

When we breathe, air flows through the windpipe (trachea) into 2 large air tubes (bronchi), then into smaller tubes (bronchioles), then to tiny air sacs (alveoli) in the lungs.

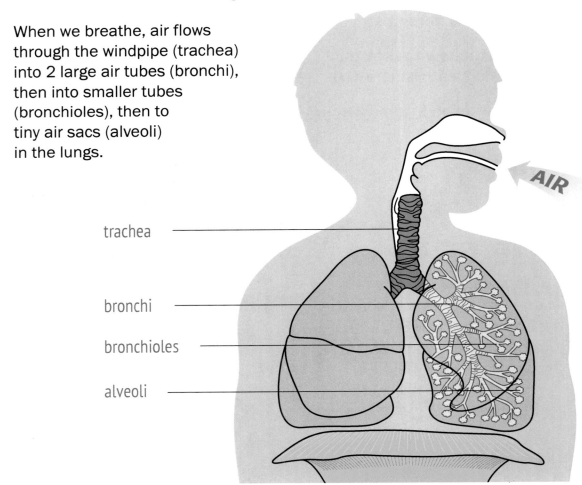

AIR

trachea

bronchi

bronchioles

alveoli

Asthma flare-ups

With asthma, your child's:

- airway muscles tighten and squeeze the airways closed

- airways swell and become inflamed, blocking the air flow

- airways make so much mucus that air cannot pass through them

During a **flare-up** (attack or episode), your child may:

- cough

- be short of breath

- have chest tightness

- wheeze (a high-pitched whistling sound of air trying to move in and out of his airways)

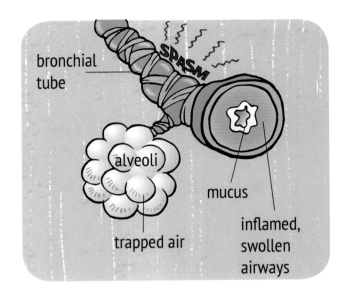

What causes a flare-up?

Things that cause asthma flare-ups are called triggers. There are many types, and they vary from child to child. Colds, flu, smoke, exercise and things he is allergic to are some of the more common triggers. Use the check list on page 8 to help you find out what your child's triggers are so you can help him avoid them. They are not always easy to spot, so it may take some time.

exercise

Most kids run and play very hard. For some children, this may trigger a flare-up. If your child feels a flare-up coming on, he should stop and rest. He may also need to take his rescue medicine.

To help **prevent a flare-up**, have him do this:

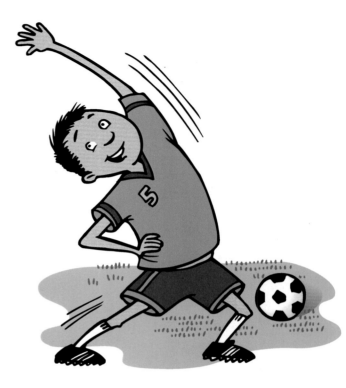

- warm up slowly, then cool down and stretch after exercise

- in cold weather, cover his mouth and nose with a scarf, muffler or ski mask (This helps warm the air before it reaches his lungs.)

- use his quick-relief medicine 15 minutes before exercise if his doctor has said to (see page 18)

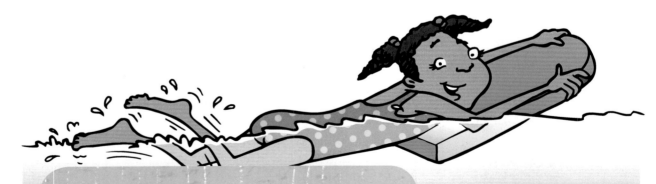

Exercise is good for your child.
With good asthma control, your child should be able to play the sports she enjoys.

allergens

Over 80% of children with asthma also have allergies to things like dust mites, molds, pollen or animals (saliva and flaking skin). These things are called *allergens*. When a child is exposed to some allergens (especially dust mites), he may have an asthma flare-up.

If you think your child may be allergic to something, talk with his doctor.

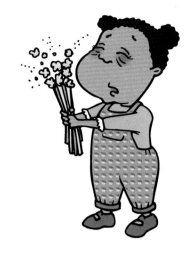

germs and infections

One of the most common triggers for children is an infection of the airways—like a cold or the flu (influenza). Flu shots are recommended for children with asthma*. Ask your doctor if your child should get a flu shot each year.

Kids pass many germs to each other by coughing, sneezing and sharing things like spoons, cups and toys. **Teach your child to wash his hands often** to avoid germs.

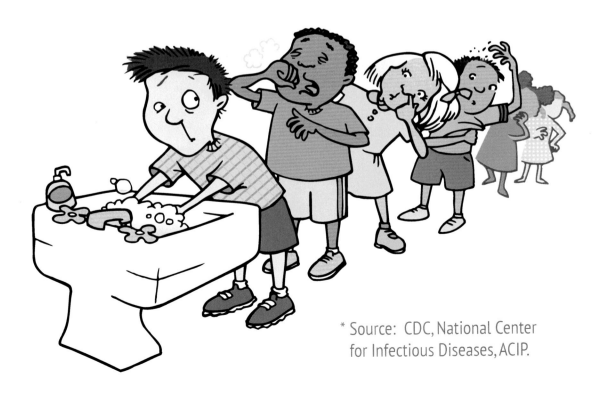

* Source: CDC, National Center for Infectious Diseases, ACIP.

dust mites

Dust mites are tiny insects that live in house dust. They are so small, you can't see them. They're very common and can trigger flare-ups when breathed into the lungs.

It's very important to control dust mites in your child's bedroom. **Make it as dust-free as you can.**

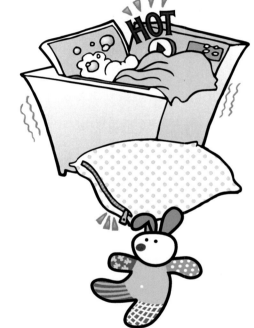

✓ Wash bed linen in hot water (130°F*) each week.

✓ Put airtight, allergy-proof, zippered covers on his pillow, box spring and mattress.

✓ Keep stuffed animals away from the bed. Avoid stuffed animals that can't be washed often in hot water (130°F*). Freezing stuffed animals for 48 hours also kills dust mites.

✓ If your child has a bunk bed, clean it well each week. If he has a bed with a canopy, wash the canopy in hot water (130°F*) each week.

✓ Clean your child's bedroom each **week.** Dust with a damp cloth. Arrange for him to be out of the room.

✓ Hardwood floors with rugs that can be washed are best for your child's bedroom. But if his room has carpet, vacuum each week, and shampoo every 3 to 4 months.

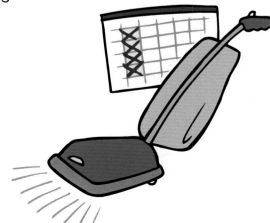

✓ Use shades instead of curtains, or wash curtains in hot water (130°F*) every month.

* At 130°F, water is very hot. So teach your family to be careful using hot water.

other ways to avoid dust mites:

✓ Give your house a **good** cleaning every three months. (Dust with a damp mop or sponge.) Arrange for your child to be out of the house when you do this. If he must be there, have him wear a dust mask.

✓ Use a vacuum with a HEPA (high-efficiency particulate arrester) filter or a double bag.

✓ Get rid of clutter that collects dust.

✓ Try a dehumidifier to keep indoor humidity below 50%. (Do not use a vaporizer daily. This will increase humidity.)

✓ Change furnace filters often (at least every three months). Change every month during winter.

✓ Cover heat vents with an air filter or cheese cloth.

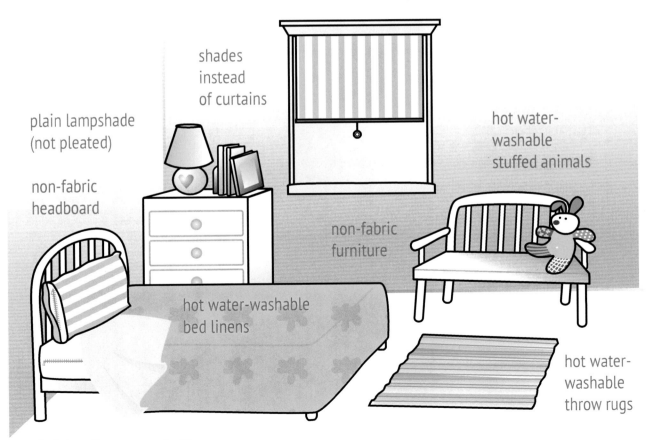

shades instead of curtains

plain lampshade (not pleated)

non-fabric headboard

hot water-washable stuffed animals

non-fabric furniture

hot water-washable bed linens

hot water-washable throw rugs

airtight, allergy-proof pillow and mattress covers

's Triggers

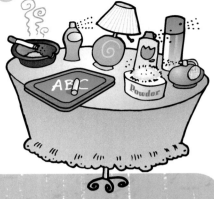

_____
child's name

Check the things that trigger your child's asthma.
Let your child check them if he can.

general irritants
(should be avoided by everyone with asthma)

- [ ] tobacco smoke
- [ ] spray deodorants, hair sprays, insect sprays, cleaning sprays
- [ ] carpet freshener, baby powder
- [ ] fragrances, perfume, cologne, scented candles, incense, Plugins®, room freshener
- [ ] chalk dust, odors from markers
- [ ] smog, pollen and other air pollution
- [ ] car and truck exhaust
- [ ] changes in temperature, humidity or air pressure
- [ ] odors from cleaning fluids, paints, furniture polish
- [ ] smoke from burning wood or leaves

Every year, secondhand smoke triggers up to 1 million asthma flare-ups in children.

others

- [ ] colds, flu, sinus problems
- [ ] exercise
- [ ] bursts of emotion that affect breathing (such as crying, laughing, etc.)
- [ ] some medicines
- [ ] _____
- [ ] _____

allergic triggers
(avoid if you are allergic to them)

- [ ] dust mites (see pages 6–7)
- [ ] cats, dogs and other furry pets
- [ ] cockroaches
- [ ] mold, mildew
- [ ] some foods (rarely)
- [ ] pollens, grass, trees, ragweed

Fish are great pets for kids with asthma— no flaking skin.

This page may be copied for your child's use.

Avoiding triggers

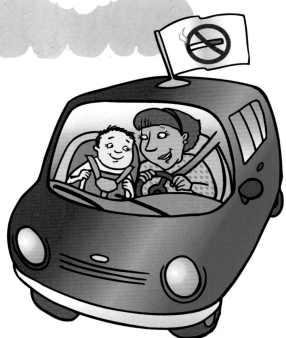

- Avoid smoke and smoky places. **Do not smoke or let anyone else ever smoke in your home or car.**

- Have your child stay away from chalk dust and use odor-free markers in school.

- Avoid air pollution! Use air-conditioning, not fans, at home. Keep windows closed. If you have air-conditioning in your car, recirculate the air or keep him inside during traffic rush hours.

- Use unscented liquid or solid products, not sprays.

- Use a stove vent to get rid of cooking fumes.

- Try to keep furry pets outdoors. Never let them in your child's bedroom. Wash bedding every week.

- Use an air cleaning device with a HEPA filter in his bedroom. Put it up on a table—not on the floor.

- Avoid mold (wet leaves, damp basements, bathrooms). Fix leaking pipes or faucets. Clean moldy surfaces.

- Use poison bait or traps to control roaches. Do not leave food or garbage out uncovered.

- Keep him away from very cold, hot or humid air.

- Don't buy foods that may cause a flare-up (foods that are triggers for **your** child). Read all food labels.

Record his asthma triggers on his asthma diary (page 26). This will help you know what to avoid in the future. If he can, let him write in his diary, too.

Treating asthma

Asthma causes more hospital stays for children than any other chronic disease. It causes more visits to the emergency room than any other childhood disease. You can prevent most of these scary events for your child. His asthma does not have to cause you to miss work or cause him to miss school. Work with his doctor to set up a **written** asthma action plan. This may include:

- learning your child's early warning signs

- avoiding triggers (see pages 4–9)

- learning what medicines to take and how to take them

With a **good asthma action plan**, your child should:

- be able to keep up with his usual activities (including exercise, sports and school)

- be free of flare-ups

- sleep through the night without waking (due to asthma)

- use a quick-relief inhaler less than 2 times a week

- have no visits to the hospital or emergency room (due to asthma)

- have few side effects from asthma medicines

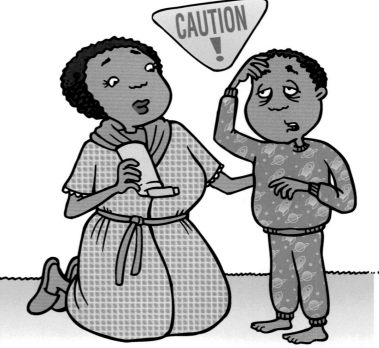

Know your child's early warning signs

An asthma flare-up begins slowly. Most children feel warning signs when a flare-up is starting. Help your child learn what his signs are and to tell you when he has them. Knowing your child's warning signs can help you and his doctor make a plan to keep a flare-up from becoming severe. Record your child's warning signs on page 14.

changes in peak flow meter scores

Your doctor may want your child to use a **peak flow meter.** (Peak flow meters may not be useful for children under the age of 5.) This is a small device that measures how well air moves out of the airways. When an asthma flare-up begins, the tiny airways of the lungs narrow slowly. **Changes in peak flow meter scores may tell you if the airways are narrowing hours or days before your child begins to cough or wheeze.** By taking medicines **early** (before other warning signs begin), you may be able to stop the flare-up quickly and prevent a severe asthma flare-up (see action plan - page 28).

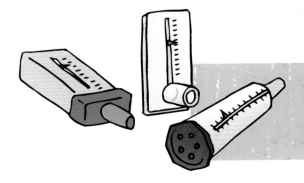

A very **early warning sign** is a **change** in peak flow meter scores.

To use a peak flow meter, have your child:

1. Stand.

2. Remove any food or gum from his mouth.

3. Slide the arrow to the bottom of the numbered scale.

4. Take a slow deep breath and blow into the peak flow meter as hard and as fast as he can. (Tell him to stop if he begins to cough or wheeze. Try again in a few minutes.)

5. Write down the number reached by the arrow.

6. Repeat steps 3–5 two more times.

7. Write down his highest score on his asthma diary—page 26. (Don't average the numbers.)

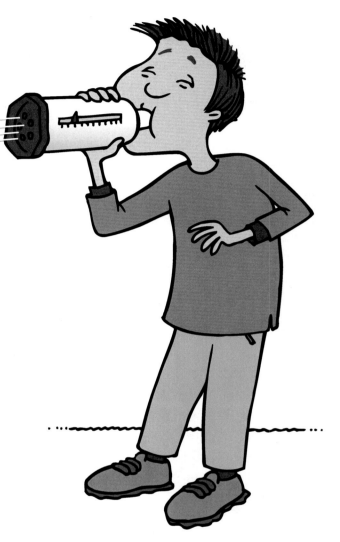

Make sure the peak flow meter is level. Your child should not blow down.

Note:
Measure his daily **peak flow meter scores** when he wakes up in the morning, before he takes his medicines.

personal best peak flow number

To use daily peak flow meter scores to check on your child's breathing, you need to have something to "check" them against. This "check" is your child's **personal best peak flow number.** This is the highest peak flow meter number he can reach when his asthma is under good control. For 2 or 3 weeks, write down his peak flow score each day. His best score during this time is his **personal best** peak flow number.

To find your child's personal best score, **measure at these times:**

- in the afternoon (between 12 noon and 2 PM may be the best time)

  or

- any other time the doctor tells you to

The doctor will use your child's personal best peak flow number—along with other early warning signs—to set up an asthma action plan.

Using your child's symptoms and his **daily** peak flow numbers, you will be able to decide if your child is in the:

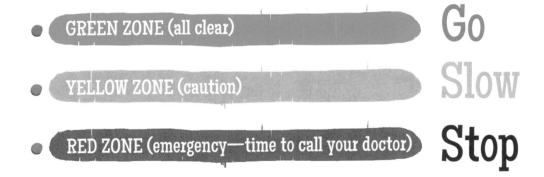

- GREEN ZONE (all clear) — Go
- YELLOW ZONE (caution) — Slow
- RED ZONE (emergency—time to call your doctor) — Stop

Using the asthma action plan on page 28, you will be able to adjust your child's treatment as needed to avoid a severe flare-up.

_____'s Warning Signs
child's name

Check the warning signs your child has had before a flare-up.

- ☐ dry cough
- ☐ stuffy nose, runny nose, watery eyes
- ☐ sneezing, itchy throat (or throat that "tickles")
- ☐ feeling tired (not wanting to "play")
- ☐ feeling sad, angry, moody or restless
- ☐ headache
- ☐ stomach ache
- ☐ ear pain
- ☐ tight chest
- ☐ wheezing
- ☐ shortness of breath or fast breathing
- ☐ trouble sleeping
- ☐ fast heartbeat
- ☐ drop in peak flow meter scores

Write in any other signs you see:

- ☐ _____
- ☐ _____
- ☐ _____
- ☐ _____

Medicines

There are two main types of asthma medicines:

- **long-term control** (preventive)

- **quick-relief** (rescue)

long-term control medicines

These are taken to prevent asthma flare-ups. Your child may have to take these for a long time. He will not become addicted even if he uses them for several years.

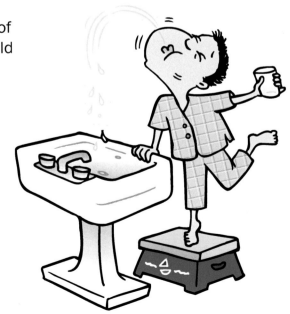

anti-inflammatory medicines

Most preventive medicines are anti-inflammatory. They help reduce swelling in the airways. Anti-inflammatories come in 2 forms: **inhaled steroid and non-steroid.**

> Your child needs to take his medicines regularly even if he feels better.

Steroid medicines are the most common type of preventive medicine. These are not the muscle-building steroids taken by some athletes. Preventive steroids are taken as a fine mist from an inhaler or a nebulizer (pages 20 and 24).

Inhaled steroids are strong medicines but are also the best medicines for long-term control of asthma. As a rule they are safe, but you should ask your child's doctor about the risk of side effects. **Your child's doctor will closely watch the use of these medicines.**

To prevent side effects (such as a sore mouth and throat or bad taste), **use with a spacer and have your child rinse his mouth with water and spit after each use** of the inhaler. If he uses a mask to inhale these medicines, have him wash his lips and face after each use.

combination medicines

Some drugs are a combination of a steroid and a long acting bronchodilator. These are usually given as an inhaler in cases of moderate to severe asthma.

This medicine is NOT a rescue inhaler!

Combination medicines include:

- Symbicort®
- Advair®
- Dulera®

The non-steroid medicines include:

- cromolyn sodium
- leukotriene modifiers
- immunomodulators

Some of these are used with an inhaler or a nebulizer and some come in pill or liquid form, or as a shot.

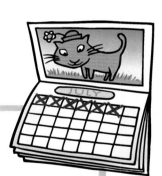

Make a note...

1. **Long-term control medicines** prevent symptoms or flare-ups by decreasing inflammation in the airways. They will not give relief for symptoms (such as wheezing, coughing, shortness of breath) your child is already showing.

2. Your child should **continue taking his long-term control medicines** even when he hasn't had any signs of asthma for several weeks or months. After his asthma has been under control for a while, your child's doctor may have you slowly decrease the amount of these medicines.

3. **Take your child's inhaler to each doctor visit.** Ask the doctor or nurse to watch your child use it and check his technique.

quick-relief medicines

When your child has an asthma flare-up, the muscle bands that open and close his airways tighten up. **Quick-relief** (rescue) medicines **relax these muscles so that air can move in and out easier.**

quick-acting inhaled bronchodilators

These are the medicines that work best for **relieving coughing, wheezing and shortness of breath.** Your child should begin to breathe easier within 10 - 30 minutes of taking his quick-relief medicine.

Quick-acting bronchodilators are breathed in (inhaled) from a hand-held inhaler (page 20) or a nebulizer (page 24). They may cause a headache, fast heart rate, trouble sleeping or jittery feeling. Most of the time, these side effects go away or get better after he has been using the medicine for a while. If they bother your child or don't improve, tell the doctor.

If exercise is one of your child's triggers, his doctor may tell you to give him one of these medicines 15 to 30 minutes before he starts to exercise.

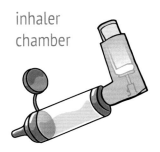
inhaler
chamber

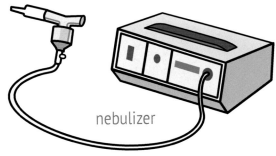
nebulizer

NOTE:
There may be times when your child will need to take these medicines every day for several days along with his preventive medicines.

CAUTION:
Never give your child any medicines (including over-the-counter medicines such as antihistamines, cough syrup and cold medicine) unless his doctor has told you it's OK.

Make a note...

1. Always have your child keep his quick-relief medicines with him at school, at home and on vacations.

2. Have him wait at least 15 to 30 seconds between puffs.

3. If he has to use his quick-relief medicine more than 2 times a week, his asthma is not in good control. His asthma action plan is not working. **Talk to his doctor** about this.

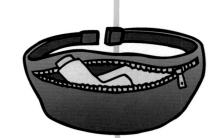

steroids (taken by pill or liquid)

Most steroids are inhaled as long-term medicines to prevent flare-ups. But if your child is in his red breathing zone, the doctor may have him take steroids as pills or liquid for several days. These are **very helpful in controlling a severe flare-up.** They may take about 4–12 hours to begin working and should be taken with food.

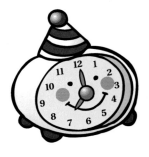

When he is taking steroids by pill or liquid, he should **continue using his inhaled preventive medicines.** He should also keep using his quick-relief medicines for fast relief of symptoms. He should never stop taking steroids without his doctor's advice.

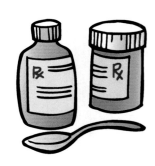

Ask the doctor to help you fill in this chart.

_____'s Medicines

child's name

Name	Type (preventive or quick-relief)	What it does	When to take	How to take	How long to take	When he will feel it working	What to do if he forgets to take	Side effects and what to do about them

This page may be copied for your child's use.

Ways to take asthma medicines

Your child may take his asthma medicine
by inhaling it, as a pill or liquid, or by injection.

inhaler

A metered dose inhaler (MDI) is a small hand-held device that allows
your child to breathe in a fine mist of medicine. The inhaler is set to
give a premeasured dose of medicine with each puff. Your doctor will
tell you how many puffs your child should take.

**To use an inhaler the right way, your child most likely needs a
spacer/holding chamber.** This will help him get the right amount
of medicine from each puff.

If your child is **5 or younger**, he may
need to use a **mask** with the spacer/holding
chamber. The doctor, nurse, pharmacist or
therapist will show your child how to use
the inhaler. Learn the steps on page 21
so you can help your child follow them.

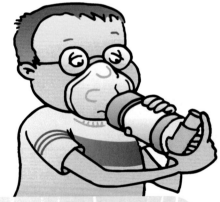

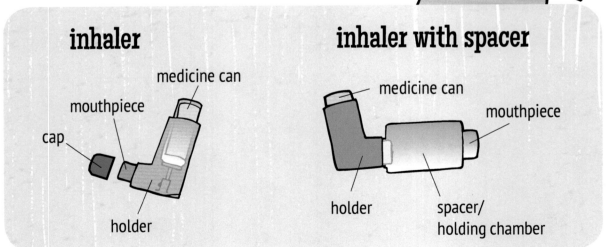

inhaler

- medicine can
- mouthpiece
- cap
- holder

inhaler with spacer

- medicine can
- mouthpiece
- holder
- spacer/ holding chamber

Some asthma medicines for older children come in a dry powder inhaler (DPI) that
releases the powder medicine into your child's mouth. Your child must then take a
deep breath to get the medicine into his lungs.

Not all inhalers or spacers are the same. Read the instructions with your package to find out exactly how your child's inhaler and spacer/holding chamber work. **For all inhalers, have your child:**

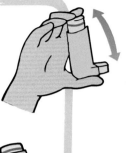

1. **Shake the inhaler well** right before each puff.

2. Prime the inhaler before first use and if it's not used every day. To prime the inhaler, hold the canister away from your face and press down to release one or more puffs.

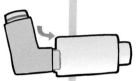

3. Remove the caps. With the inhaler in the upright position, insert the mouthpiece of the inhaler into the spacer or holding chamber.

4. Stand or sit up straight and, when ready, gently breathe out.

5. Put the mouthpiece of the spacer/holding chamber into his mouth—**over the tongue** and between the teeth. Seal his lips around the mouthpiece. If he is using a mask with a spacer, **place the mask snugly over his nose and mouth.**

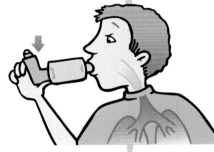

6. Start to slowly breathe in, then press down on the metal can to release 1 puff of the medicine.

7. **Breathe in slowly** and **deeply** to fill the lungs. If he is using a mask, hold it in place and have him take at least **6 breaths.**

8. Have him **hold his breath** for 10 seconds and then breathe out slowly while keeping his lips sealed on the mouthpiece.

9. If he is supposed to take more than one puff, repeat steps 4–8. For the **quick-relief meds**, wait 15 to 30 seconds between puffs to let the first puff begin working.

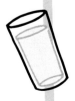

10. When he's finished, have him **rinse** his mouth **and spit** (not needed when using quick-relief).

11. Follow the directions on the package to clean and store the inhaler and spacer.

CAUTION:
The contents of an inhaler are under pressure. Don't let your child keep it or use it near an open flame.

don't run out

It's hard to tell when an inhaler is empty. All inhalers will continue to spray air (propellant) after the medicine is gone.

If your inhaler does not have a counter, one way to tell if the inhaler is empty is to make a chart. Follow these steps:

1. **Look at the number of puffs** on the side of the medicine can. ("Inhalations" means "puffs.") Write that number down.

2. **Write down the date and how many puffs** your child takes each time (include "puffs" used for priming).

3. **Add the numbers** in the total column each week to see how close you are to the total number of puffs in the inhaler.

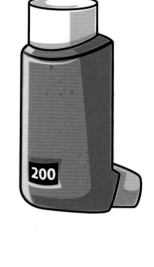

If using a chart is not handy, you or your child can make a mark on the medicine can or the inhaler box each time he takes a puff. Then you can add up the marks at the end of each week.

You can also use an inhaler counter to keep track of the number of puffs. You can find these at asthma and allergy supply centers.

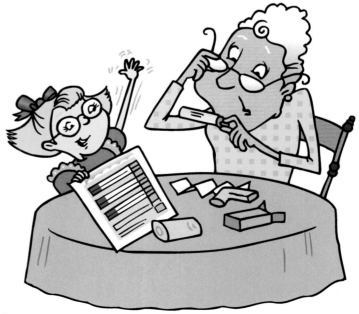

Make sure you prime your inhaler the first time you use it and again if you haven't used it for several days.

To prime your inhaler:

- Take the cap off and shake the inhaler.

- Spray a puff of medicine away from your face.

- Shake and spray the inhaler like this 2-4 more times.

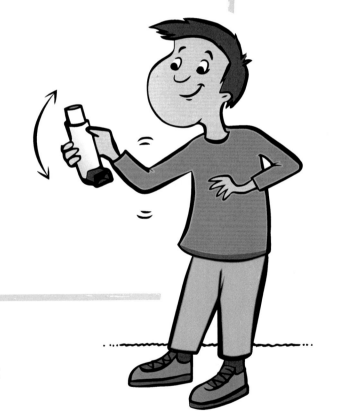

Different medicines have different priming instructions.

Check with your pharmacist or on the package label for exact priming instructions for your device.

nebulizer

With a nebulizer, your child breathes
a fine mist of medicine into his lungs.
The medicine is breathed in through
a mask or mouthpiece.

Depending on your child's age and
asthma action plan, a nebulizer may be used:

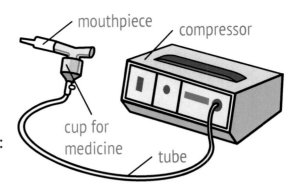

nebulizer

- during a severe flare-up

- when your child has trouble using the inhaler

When your child uses a nebulizer:

- Make sure the doctor or company that supplies
  you with the nebulizer shows you how to use it.

- Follow the doctor's orders when adding medicine.

- Clean the parts of the nebulizer according to the directions
  that come with the machine.

- Write down the name and phone number of the company
  that sold you the nebulizer in case you have problems.

CAUTION:

- Medicine made for a nebulizer
  can be **very harmful** (even
  cause death) **if he drinks it.**
- Be careful with medicines
  around young children.
- Your child should take
  medicine only as his
  doctor tells him to.

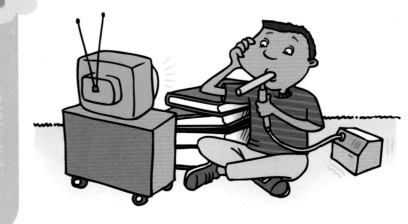

Asthma diary: putting it all together

The asthma diary on the next page will help you and your doctor:

- learn what makes your child's asthma worse
- decide if his asthma action plan is working
- know when to add or stop a medicine
- decide when to get emergency help

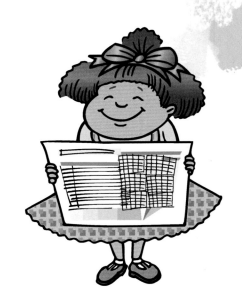

To make the diary most useful:

1. Fill it in **every** day. It's hard to remember what happened if you skip 2 or 3 days.

2. Let your child help fill it in. This will help him learn what's important to tell you.

3. Take it to every doctor visit.

4. Remind the doctor that you would like to talk about it.

5. Save the completed diaries for several months. These will help you know what's needed for long-term asthma control.

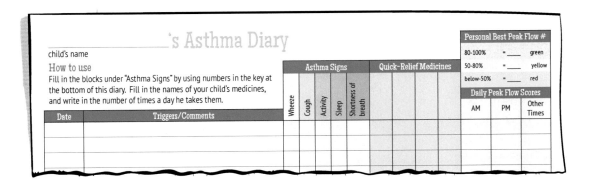

_____'s Asthma Diary

child's name _____

How to use

Fill in the blocks under "Asthma Signs" by using numbers in the key at the bottom of this diary. Fill in the names of your child's medicines, and write in the number of times a day he takes them.

Personal Best Peak Flow #		
80-100%	= _____	green
50-80%	= _____	yellow
below-50%	= _____	red

Daily Peak Flow Scores

	AM	PM	Other Times

Date	Triggers/Comments	Asthma Signs					Quick-Relief Medicines				Daily Peak Flow Scores		
		Wheeze	Cough	Activity	Sleep	Shortness of breath					AM	PM	Other Times

Wheeze

- None = 0
- Occasional = 1
- Frequent = 2
- Continuous = 3

Cough

- None = 0
- Occasional = 1
- Frequent = 2
- Continuous = 3

Activity

- Normal = 0
- Can run short distance = 1
- Can walk only = 2
- Missed school or stayed indoors = 3

Sleep

- Fine = 0
- Slept well, slight wheeze or cough = 1
- Awake 2 – 3 times, wheeze or cough = 2
- Bad night, awake most of the time = 3

Shortness of breath

- Fine = 0
- Slept well, slight wheeze or cough = 1
- Awake 2 – 3 times, wheeze or cough = 2
- Bad night, awake most of the time = 3

Adapted with permission from National Asthma Education and Prevention Program, Expert Panel Report 2, National Institutes of Health

Working with the doctor

You, your child and his doctor must work together to find the asthma action plan that works best. Ask his doctor how often your child should visit. To get the most from these visits:

- **Keep your dates.** Remind yourself of his visits. Put notes on your refrigerator, calendar or dresser.

- **Take his inhalers, peak flow meter and asthma diary with you.** Show the doctor how he uses these.

- **Ask questions.** Write them down before the doctor visit. Be sure you understand the doctor's answers.

- **Give information.** Have your child tell his doctor how he has felt since his last visit. Share his diary and peak flow meter scores. Talk about how and when he takes his medicines.

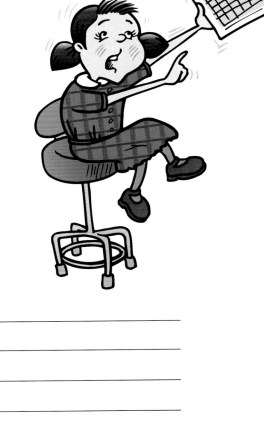

- **Follow directions.** Write down everything the doctor tells you, and follow your child's written asthma action plan closely.

Questions for the doctor:

_____

_____

_____

_____

_____

Personal Best Peak Flow Meter Score_____

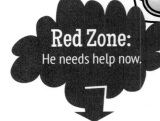

_____'s Asthma Action Plan

child's name

Green Zone:
He is breathing his best.

He:

- has peak flow meter scores greater than _____ (80% of his personal best peak flow number)
- sleeps through the night without coughing or wheezing
- has no early warning signs of an asthma flare-up
- can do usual activities

Take preventive medicines:

- _____
- _____
- _____
- _____

Continue to avoid triggers.

Take quick-relief medicines 15 minutes before exercise.

- _____
- _____
- _____
- _____

Yellow Zone:
He is not breathing his best.

He may:

- have a peak flow meter score between ___ – ___ (50%–80% of his personal best peak flow number)
- be coughing or wheezing at night
- have early warning signs of a flare-up
- have trouble doing his usual activities (school, play, exercise)

Take quick-relief medicines:

- _____
- _____

Continue or increase preventive medicines.

- _____
- _____

Call his doctor if:

- he stays in the yellow zone for more than ____ hours
- his symptoms are getting worse
- he uses his quick-relief medicine more often than every 4 hours or ____ times a day

Red Zone:
He needs help now.

He may:

- have a peak flow meter score less than_____ (50% of his personal best peak flow number)
- be coughing, short of breath, wheezing
- suck in skin between ribs, above his breastbone and collarbone when breathing
- have trouble walking or talking

Emergency Medicine Plan:

- take quick-relief medicine
- _____
- _____
- _____

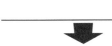

Call your doctor or emergency room and ask what to do.

Call 911 if:

- his nails or lips are blue
- he has trouble walking or talking
- he cannot stop coughing

Take the Asthma Control Test (ACT):
Google "asthma control test" for various examples.

This page may be copied for your child's use.

When to call the doctor

Ask your child's doctor to check the signs below that tell you when to call him or her.

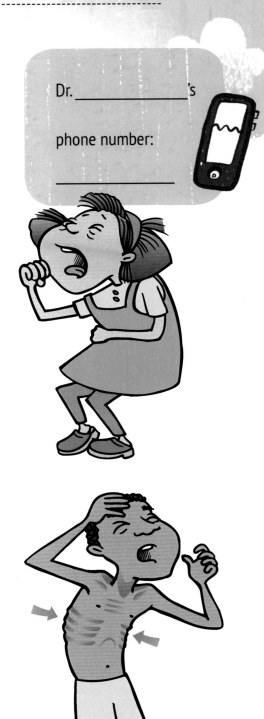

Dr. _____'s

phone number:

_____

- ☐ wheezing that does not get better after using quick-relief medicines

- ☐ using quick-relief medicines more than every 4 hours or 4 times a day

- ☐ hard coughing, too much mucus

- ☐ coughing that keeps your child up at night

- ☐ cannot stop coughing

- ☐ missing activities often (such as school, play) due to asthma

- ☐ rapid breathing

- ☐ shortness of breath

- ☐ breathing so hard that the skin between the ribs, above the breastbone and above the collarbone pulls in

- ☐ chest tightness

- ☐ weakness, trouble exercising, weak voice, can't speak in sentences

- ☐ low peak flow meter scores that do not improve after taking relief medicine

Working with the teacher

Your child's teacher (and other adults who care for him) should be aware of his needs. It's a good idea to give his teacher a copy of the written asthma action plan and the "When to call the doctor" page. Go over the plan with his teacher. Then ask if there are any questions about what to do in case of a flare-up.

Tell adults who care for your child to **trust him** when he tells them how he feels. Your child knows his body and asthma symptoms better than anyone else.

Your child may need a permission form to take medicine to school. Use the letter on the next page or create your own. If he is showing symptoms before he leaves, send a note to school so he can skip gym class. Ask that he stays calm at recess. If exercise is a trigger, give him quick-relief medicines 15 to 20 minutes before gym or recess.

When to keep your child home

When your child is having asthma problems, it may not be a good idea for him to leave home. Have him stay home if he:

- has trouble breathing even after taking his medicine

- gets winded when speaking or just playing quietly

- cannot stop coughing

- was up at night due to coughing

- is in his yellow zone after taking **quick-relief medicine**

- quick-relief medicine is needed more often than every 4 hours or more than 4 times a day

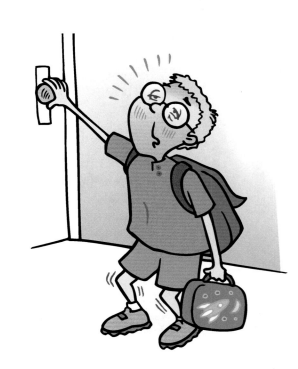

Sample School Letter

Dear _____,

My child, _____, born _____, has asthma.

My child's asthma action plan includes taking medicine with a Metered Dose Inhaler (MDI). Instructions for using an MDI:

1. Store at room temperature.

2. Shake the MDI for 5 seconds before each use.

3. Prime the MDI before the first use or when not used every day. Follow the product's patient information sheet for MDI specific priming instructions. Priming usually involves pressing down on the medication canister to discard into the air one or more puffs of medication. Discarding puffs makes sure the next puff inhaled contains the labeled amount of mediation.

4. If the inhaler does not have a counter, keep track of metered inhalation puffs used. Subtract the number used from the number of metered inhalation puffs available listed on the label. The number of metered inhaled puffs available is listed on the medication canister or on the box. There are usually 120 or 200 puffs in an MDI.

5. Ask family for a new MDI **before** all labeled metered inhalation puffs are used.

Please allow time for my child to do this if it is needed.

There is the possibility of a reaction to the MDI and medicine. Symptoms include headache, shakiness, fast heart rate, nausea. Please call me if symptoms increase in intensity or interfere with schoolwork and activity; or if MDI usage is frequent (more than every 4 hours).

My name _____

My work number _____

My home number _____

My cell number _____

My child's doctor's name _____

Doctor's office number _____

Asthma on the go

Your child must always keep his inhaler and quick-relief medicines nearby. If he goes on a trip or spends the night out, he must be even more prepared. Make a checklist to be sure he is ready before he leaves. If you travel by air, make sure you take medicine and supplies on the plane.

_____'s Travel Checklist
child's name

Medicines

- [ ] enough medicine for vacation, plus some extra
- [ ] a list of all medicines
- [ ] labels from pharmacy bottles (for emergency refills)
- [ ] medicines and inhaler with spacer and/or mask

Equipment

- [ ] peak flow meter
- [ ] nebulizer and supplies, if needed
- [ ] anti-dust mite items, if needed (pillow and mattress covers)
- [ ] medical alert bracelet or necklace, if needed
- [ ] fanny pack to carry supplies

Records

- [ ] treatment plan
- [ ] asthma diary with peak flow meter numbers
- [ ] medical insurance card(s)
- [ ] doctor's phone number
- [ ] names of asthma specialists where your child is going

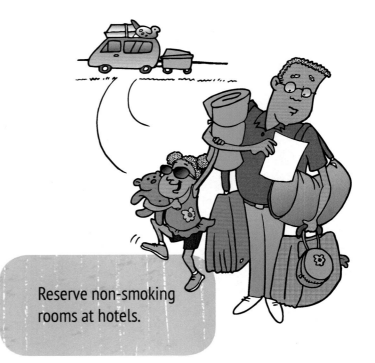

Reserve non-smoking rooms at hotels.

Resources

These groups want to help you and your child manage his asthma. They can answer questions and send information. Most of the information is free.

- **Allergy and Asthma Network**
  1-800-878-4403
  aanma.org

- **American Academy of Allergy, Asthma and Immunology**
  aaaai.org

- **American College of Allergy, Asthma and Immunology**
  1-847-427-1200
  acaai.org

- **American Lung Association**
  1-800-586-4872
  lung.org

- **Asthma Control Test (ACT)**
  Google "asthma control test"

- **Asthma & Allergy Foundation of America (AAFA)**
  1-800-727-8462
  aafa.org
  e-mail: info@aafa.org

- **Lung Line, National Jewish Medical & Research Center**
  1-800-222-LUNG
  (222-5864)
  nationaljewish.org

- **National Institute of Allergy and Infectious Diseases**
  1-301-496-5717
  www.niaid.nih.gov

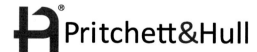

Pritchett&Hull

PRITCHETT & HULL ASSOCIATES, INC.

bringing Patients & Health together since 1973

Limited list of topics include:

Write or call toll-free for a free catalog of all products and prices at **1-800-241-4925** or visit P&H online at **www.p-h.com**

Made in the USA
Middletown, DE
05 November 2016